Freedom Thru Fitness

Freedom Thru Fitness

by

Matthew Sinosky

White Publishing | Norwell, MA

Publisher: White Publishing, Norwell, MA
Editor: Steve White

Cover: Photograph by W. James King (Henry's Studio)

First Edition: June 2017

Printed in the United States of America

ISBN: 978-0-692-89888-8

Dedication

To My Wife, Lindsey, my kids, Mattison and Chase, and all the friends and family who have given me support throughout the years. Thank you all!

Table of Contents

Introduction

Thanks for taking the time to pick up my book. I know how busy you are so let me save you some time that might be better spent doing something else. All you have to do is answer one simple question:

Are you happy with your body?

If you answered "yes," that's fine. Put down this book, head for the gym, run a marathon, subscribe to one of those muscle magazines. You have accomplished something truly remarkable, and for that I commend you and encourage you to keep it up!

But if you answered "no," then you are one of those many people who seem to constantly struggle to maintain a consistent workout regimen, find that perfect diet, be happy with your appearance, or do simple physical activities in order to improve your overall health. In fact, the majority of our population falls into this category. It is estimated that approximately two thirds of the adult population in the United States is considered overweight. By my own estimation, this seems pretty accurate. Have you ever gone to the beach and really looked around at the people out there?

Sadly, I was one of those people. It wasn't too long ago I was 50 lbs heavier and trending upwards. I had terrible eating and drinking habits. I had no regular exercise regimen. Okay, let's be honest....I was straight up lazy and lacked any sort of ambition or discipline. Hey, at least I wasn't in denial. I knew I was fat. My wife knew I was fat (but because she loves me she wouldn't come right out and say it). My doctor knew I was fat (well, he actually *did* come out and say it). I ate too much, drank too much and felt sluggish and tired all the time. I was diagnosed with sleep apnea, which was in direct relation to my weight. I was becoming a mess.

So I made a decision once my wife and I had our second child to get serious and get healthy. I wanted to be a better example for my wife and kids. I educated myself by looking at diet and exercise books and magazines. I spent countless number of hours reading and researching on how to eat and how to exercise. I looked into several different programs that I could purchase and follow, but none gave me the feeling that their program would be the long-term answer for me. So after months of research I made the decision to tackle this problem on my own.

Over the years I tried many different things and what I discovered along the way was that most of the exercise plans out there are not built for long-term sustainability. They have a defined duration and as such always lead you to a less than optimal end because they don't offer you any continuity, which is why I decided to do things my own way. My philosophy is to mix in elements of various workout routines, but to do so in an independent manner so there is no end and you can continue your fit lifestyle indefinitely, without help from any outside sources and without subscribing to a specific program.

I am going to share with you what I learned along the way and what actually works in real life, not just in the pages of some magazine or the latest, hottest self-help book. I want to be very clear from the start that there is NOTHING spectacular about me other than the fact that I have been able to maintain discipline in both my eating and exercise. There are a lot of people out there who are bigger, stronger, faster, built better, and dedicate more time and resources to their fitness, but I often feel those people aren't the best example of fitness for the average person. I think most people look at individuals like that and become defeated right out of the gate because they don't feel they can ever get there and, in most cases, they are right. People who are exceedingly muscular with low body fat are not only taking a tremendous amount of supplements and putting in a tremendous amount of work, but they are also genetically blessed. On the other hand, me, I am simply a guy who was overweight, out of shape, and went through all of this on my own and got some decent results which anybody could achieve if they put in the time and effort. I am not some certified physical trainer, or a physician with numerous degrees, or some incredible beast in the gym. I did it by experimenting and picking up information along the way. And once I dropped the 50 lbs, I decided I wanted to share how I did it with average people just like me. I wanted people to feel the satisfaction I felt every time I stepped on a scale, looked in a mirror, or tackled a new physical challenge that I could accomplish with no issue.

The bottom line is this: everyone is capable of reaching a level of fitness that will have you happy with your body, your physical abilities, and how you feel. We can't control our genetics; we can only control our diet, our workout, and the effort we put forth in each.

I have learned through self-education that most people who struggle with their weight or fitness level simply lack the direction, focus, and, most importantly, the discipline to reach and maintain certain goals. This book will show you the methods that have worked for me, methods that are effective and sustainable for obtaining long-term results. Sadly, most people focus on short-term goals and once reached they revert to their normal activity. My goal is to teach you through my own personal experience how to *make and reach long-term goals* that will change your entire lifestyle.

In this book we will cover from start to finish the steps you need to take in order to change your life. You will have at your fingertips the basic principles to guide you, but also the flexibility to change up your routine within those guiding principles to suit your needs. And it doesn't matter if you are a man or woman, old or young. If you follow these basics principles and build on them you will get results. And best of all, you will no longer be held hostage by your own body. This book will be your key to total physical freedom.

I want you to keep in mind that this book is not focused on a specific area nor is it an exact plan to follow. My goal in providing this information is that you will have a road map, guiding principles, to living a fit lifestyle. My plan can certainly be modified in order to achieve certain strengths above others. For example, if, in addition to fitness, your goal is endurance for distance running then your workout plan will be heavier on the running and cardio while someone who prefers to be bigger or stronger would focus on weight training. However, if your goal is to get to 3% body fat, break marathon records, or bench 500 lbs, my plan will most likely not get you there.

But if you want to be fit overall and maybe focus on being a *little* bigger, a *little* stronger, a *little* faster, or a *little* leaner than the average guy, then my plan is for you and you'll be happy you picked up this book. Let's begin.

Chapter 1

Making a Lifestyle Choice

If you are taking the time out of your busy day to read this book, then you have already made the choice to improve your lifestyle. That's good. Because even if you can't control everything in your life, you *can* control the type of lifestyle you want to live. Making the choice to change your lifestyle to one that is active and revolves around fitness is the key to making your fitness sustainable. By embracing fitness in your lifestyle you will develop a passion for it and it's important that you remain passionate about what you are doing. If you are not passionate you will have a difficult time sticking with your plan. I don't mean that you need to be passionate about your workout or your diet, but you *do* need to be passionate about your goals and how you want to live your life. Your workout and diet are simply a means to that end. That is why this step is so important. It is easy to lose your passion to work out because you don't have time

1

or don't feel well, but you should *never* lose your passion to live the life you want. If you do lose that passion, then you have bigger problems than I can solve in this book.

Before we go on, I want to clarify that when I talk about lifestyle I am not referring to lifestyle in the sense of being rich and famous. I am referring to your level of activity in your life and how you feel-- your physical lifestyle. My approach takes little or no money, so your financial situation is no excuse. As we go through the various stages of my approach I will detail examples of variations on my nutrition, workout plan, and supplementation to show that it can all be done without costing you a lot of money. I understand that money is an issue for a lot of people and they will use that as an excuse. When I started my path to fitness eight years ago I was making $40,000 per year, just bought a house, and couldn't justify dropping $1,000 per year on a gym membership and supplements. I bought a Bowflex for $200 on eBay and relied on that for my resistance training and ran to increase my cardio. I didn't take any supplements because I couldn't afford them. Choosing and living an active lifestyle can be done no matter your financial position. The only things in your way are excuses.

We often look at others who are active and think, "I wish I could do that." Well stop wishing and start doing! The truth is that you are likely capable of doing 99% of what you see others doing if you are willing to commit the time and effort it takes to do those things. When people say, "I wish I could play the guitar, rock climb, run a marathon, write a book, etc.", that isn't exactly what they mean. What they are actually saying is, "I wish I had the commitment and the drive to do those things." The truth is if you really wanted to play the guitar then you would get lessons and practice until you could play. If you wanted to be a rock climber or run a marathon or write a book, you would do the same. I hate hearing these statements. If you wish you could do something, then go and do it! People like to say they wish they could do things because saying it is a lot easier than actually going out and doing it. Getting in shape is no different. You start off saying you want to get in shape and you do it for a while and see some quick results. But then the weight losses or muscle gains start to level off and you get discouraged. Getting in shape, losing weight, building muscle takes time and effort period, but it can be done. If you say you want to get in shape be patient and do it.

I have discovered that there is generally a very small margin between the natural capabilities people possess. The differentiator is how much time, effort, and commitment those who are active put in to achieve the abilities they want. There is nothing limiting you in what you're a capable of doing except your desire to do it. If you want something you have to commit the time and energy to get what you want. There is very little that comes naturally for people. While genetics can help us out, they are not the ultimate determining factor in how we look or what we can do. So don't use your genetics as an excuse to prevent yourself from reaching your goals.

Be someone who is a "doer" not a talker. I tend to be both. I talk in order to drive myself a bit to do things. I have an absolute fear of failure......I hate the prospect of it, and so should you. Take this book, for example, when I decided I was going to write a book I told everyone about it (I talked) before even beginning and I told them when it would be finished. These set expectations that if I did not reach would be a failure in the eyes of many people who were important to me. I did the same thing when I decided I was going to start running 5Ks, mud races, half-marathons, etc. I told people I was going to do it which set me up for failure if I didn't do it. A constant theme throughout this book is to develop a hatred for failure and avoid it at all costs! Any great competitor will tell you that they hate losing more than they love winning. This is exactly why this planning stage is so important and we need to set expectations that are a stretch but are achievable so when we reach them we don't celebrate too much, but when we miss them is feels like a failure. Avoid failure at all costs. The more times you accept failure, the easier it will be to accept!

Making the decision about what you want out of your life will be the driver in everything that we talk about. Your decision about lifestyle will go hand-in-hand with your goals, which will lead to your workout/nutrition plan and your execution of that plan.

When making your lifestyle choice you need to think about things like:

1) How do I want to live?
2) What do I want to look like?
3) What do I want to be capable of doing?
4) What kind of activity level do I want to have?

If you can answer these questions *honestly*, you will have a good guide to deciding the lifestyle that you want to live. It will also help you to understand and accept the commitment that it will take to sustain that lifestyle. You do not have to accept how you are currently living. Your lifestyle is a conscious choice that you will make and be responsible for achieving. Regardless of how you answer these questions, and the lifestyle you decide that you want, you need to drop the "I can't" attitude and take responsibility for how you choose to live. Often times the only thing in the way of your goals is yourself. So get out of your way and get going!

There are many choices we can make in terms of our lifestyle. We can choose to be:

1) Sedentary
2) Unhealthy
3) Overweight
4) Lazy
5) Inactive
6) Hardworking
7) Fit
8) Active
9) Adventurous
10) Inspired
11) Competitive

If you want to live the lifestyle mapped out in choices one through five, then you picked up the wrong book. Perhaps Amazon has one titled, "Why I Want to Be a Loser." But if you are ready to change, work hard and get fit, then you've come to the right place. Like I said, anyone can change their lifestyle. We all certainly have physical limitations based on our genetics, but we can ALL make drastic changes in the way we live no matter our genetic predisposition. Whether you are 6'8 and 150 lbs, or 4'8 and 400 lbs, you can make a decision to change and execute it through a good plan, hard work, and discipline.

Chapter 2

Goal Setting

Goal setting is extremely important and probably the most overlooked aspect of any type of plan. It's not just about working out or losing weight. Anything we seek to accomplish requires planning and the establishment of defined goals. Most people simply start down the path of working on something and try to do the best they can, but without goals there are no markers to gauge their progress and, more importantly, the effectiveness of their workout.

Make your goals incremental and achievable. If you set goals that are too lofty you will get overwhelmed trying to reach those goals and will become discouraged by the amount of time it may take you to reach them... if you reach them at all. You want to push yourself in your workout and nutrition plan, but you also want to avoid failure. Make your goals realistic and attainable, so they require you to work hard in order to achieve them. Even the smallest of failures may discourage you from continuing on your journey toward a fit lifestyle. If your goals are set with some thought and purpose, and you know they are achievable if you push yourself outside of your comfort zone, chances are you will avoid failure at all costs to get to that goal. Look to constantly push yourself out of your comfort zone. Being uncomfortable is a good thing. Growth in life comes outside the comfort zone.

Establish your goals with *you* in mind. Don't compare yourself to other people in terms of strength or build. Everyone is going to have different capabilities and body types so just strive for continuous improvement for yourself. Aim to be happy with yourself, not in comparison to others.

There are some that feel that you should set extremely high goals, so if you fall short you still achieve great gains. You have probably heard the expression, "Shoot for the stars and if you miss you'll still hit the moon." I have a problem with this because if you are as determined as I am then you will not accept failure in achieving those goals. For example, if your goal is to bench press 500 lbs that is A.) unattainable for most people and B.) if you do have the physiology to actually do that it will take all of your commitment and effort to get there which takes your focus off your overall goal of a fit lifestyle that is sustainable. If the goals are seemingly unreachable it will have just the opposite effect; you will accept failure very quickly and give up on that goal. You should avoid falling into this trap in both your life and fitness goals. Set incremental goals and adjust them as you hit them; constantly resetting and targeting better results or new areas of improvement. Your goals should make you reach, but not overextend.

When I started this journey I weighed 240 lbs, which doesn't seem like much, but for my six-foot frame and my body fat % at the time that was a sloppy weight for me. My first goal was to get to 215 lbs. It took me six months to drop that weight, which I accomplished by improving my eating habits and undertaking moderate exercise. When I hit that goal I looked at my body, determined how I felt, and then decided that I wanted to get to 200 lbs, but no further. When I hit my goal of 200 lbs, I readjusted my goals to focus on other areas. Cardio has always been a challenge for me as I have always hated running, but I set out to start running some 5Ks, with the goal of finishing in the 20-21 minute range. That was in 2011, and hitting that initial goal helped me maintain a running routine to this day. My goals now are more focused on body composition and strength as I have improved my appearance and fitness, keeping my weight consistently between 190 and 200 lbs.

I started out with a weight goal because I had a lot of excess weight to lose, but I always caution people not to get hung up on the number on the scale. If you are under 40 years of age and new to weight training, chances are that you are going to add muscle mass which weighs more than fat, so the net effect on your scale may be minimal. You need to know your body if you are going to set your goals by weight. Again, if you have a lot of excess weight to lose, then starting with a weight goal is fine. However, if weight isn't an issue for you and you are just looking to tone up (increasing muscle and decreasing body fat), then your goals will need to be different. You may need to take the approach that I do now, where your goals are set around body composition or fitness goals, such as zeroing in on cardiovascular or strength targets you want to hit. You can also use measurements like waist, chest, hip, or arm size to monitor your progress. Although my weight hasn't fluctuated outside of that 10-lb range (190-200) in the last six or seven years, my body structure has changed completely. I am a lot leaner now and a lot broader. Over the last year I have dropped two inches in my pants size and haven't lost a pound. This is because I have leaned up and increased the muscles in my chest, shoulders, back, and legs. Instead of looking at a scale to measure your progress just look in the mirror, at the weight you are lifting, or monitor how you feel as you continue to push your cardio limits. These will be much better markers for you on your progress than the scale.

In order to be great in one area it takes extreme dedication and there is something to be said for that in many areas of your life. For fitness, however, at least for the average person, there is a need for a more well-rounded approach. What kind of shape are you really in if you can run a marathon in three hours, but you can't bench press half your body weight? Or if you can bench 500 lbs, but don't have the stamina to run around the block. Keep this in mind as you set your goals. You want to focus on overall fitness. There is certainly room to enhance your performance in a specific area, but you don't want to neglect other areas of your regimen.

My goals and workout plan are heavy on weight training, but I never neglect the cardio portion of my workout. I want to make sure that I maintain a certain level of cardio fitness and fat burning activities. It can be very easy to get caught up in the things you like to do the most in the gym and neglect the things that make you uncomfortable. The truth is that the activities that make you uncomfortable are the ones that will lead you to the biggest gains. The reason for this is that activities or exercises that make you uncomfortable do so because they are difficult, signifying that they are hitting your areas of weakness and, subsequently, will provide you with the biggest opportunity for gain.

In my case, I was your average, everyday weight lifter (benching, working some back and arms) and I always avoided doing Olympic weightlifting movements like power cleans, snatches, dead lifts, squats, etc. Recently, I started committing a full workout in my cycle (on my leg day) to doing those types of exercises. I have been amazed by the results. My leg strength has gone through the roof and my core really tightened up. Now I look forward to that day in my workout because I know it is going to give me results. Even though I still dread the movements and lifts, I am driven by the result. Force yourself in every workout to incorporate a few exercises that make you really uncomfortable……you will not regret it! You will see more gains in life by doing things that are uncomfortable than you will be sticking to things you are comfortable doing. Put this to the test in all aspects of your life and make note of the results.

My approach will be effective, but it is important that you are disciplined and constantly evaluating your achievements, adjusting your goals, and setting goals in new areas so you always have targets to hit and points to measure. I am not a fan of taking time to celebrate your goals. Remember we are setting incremental goals, so hitting them isn't a lifetime achievement. When you hit your goal set a new one and get right to it. If you are someone who needs to be rewarded when you hit your goals, then you are going to struggle to sustain a diet or workout plan because you will take a break to reward yourself. You need to break yourself of that mentality before you set your goals and be prepared to be disciplined and drive through your list of goals. Never be satisfied or content when you hit a new goal in your fitness or in your life, for that matter. Once you reach a level of contentment then all progress will cease. Strive for continuous improvement and don't lose that desire to want more!

Chapter 3

Fitness Isn't Easy, Quick, or Fun....So Get Over It!

Fitness isn't easy, quick, or fun. If it were the majority of people in this country wouldn't be overweight and out of shape. Unfortunately, people gravitate toward things that are easy to do, quickly satisfying, and fun in the process, so something that isn't easy, quick, or fun doesn't scratch that itch.

I think the mistake most people make when trying to get into a workout routine is that they feel they need to find something that is one of these things – easy, quick, fun, or some combination of the three. This mentality is supported by all the programs you see developed and advertised that promote fitness; they claim to be easy, quick, or fun. For the most part, fitness is none of these things. As I pointed out in the previous chapter, my first goal was to drop 25 lbs and it took me over six months of hard work. It wasn't easy, quick, or fun. But sustainable fitness takes *time* and *effort*.

Easy Fitness

Sure it sounds like an oxymoron, but there are a lot of programs out there which advertise "easy fitness." You see ads pitching abs machines, electronic devices, magnetic devices, ab toning belts, weight loss supplements, diet plans, all promising to show how easy it is to get fit and lose weight. While some of these gadgets, supplements, or programs may help, none of them are effective on their own. And even then, they are only minimally effective unless coupled with proper diet and exercise. Nothing in life worth doing is easy. Getting a college degree, building your career, getting married, having and raising children, none of these things are easy, in fact, they are some of the most challenging things you will ever do in your life. But they are also the most rewarding. Fitness falls right in there with those things. There is only one way to stay fit and that is through hard work and discipline. It is very tempting to buy into some of the things that are advertised out there because we are all working hard at other things in our life and when we see things advertised that will give us quick results with minimal work, people will tend to gravitate toward that. An *easier method* is tempting, but do not get sucked into this trap.

Quick Fitness

Nothing sustainable or long term will be executed quickly. You don't get rock hard abs in seven minutes. You don't get fit in 90 days... then stay fit forever. Workout machines that advertise all you need is 20 minutes a day to get fit are offering false promises. You aren't going to get the results you want without putting in the extra effort and supplementing that effort with weight training or some other activity. Do you really think those people modeling on fitness product infomercials got those physiques by doing a 20 minute a day workout? Do not be fooled by what you see on TV. What you see is only a single element of what it would take to achieve a high level of fitness. Fitness takes time.

Fun Fitness

I need to be careful here because some fitness can be fun. I engage in several activities that are great fun and I incorporate them into my overall workout routine, such as CrossFit, playing

17

hockey, mountain biking, Brazilian Jiu-Jitsu, Muay Thai, running, hiking, and hunting. While fun activities can be part of your workout, this cannot be the sole basis. The majority of your workout should be intense resistance training, which for the average person is not fun, but most definitely necessary to push you forward. So the basis for your workout shouldn't be 'fun'. Still, if possible, you should supplement your core routine with whatever you deem to be fun activities. I weight train and do some form of cardio every day. Some days it is a strict workout where I am doing some form of cardio, such as running, stair-climbing, rowing, or weight training. On days when I am going to be practicing Jiu-Jitsu, playing hockey, or hunting along some tough terrain I will skip the cardio portion of my organized workout. Instead, I will just do the weight training and substitute the activity for the cardio.

Keep in mind that while your workout isn't fun the final result is fun. Looking good is fun. Feeling good is fun. Being healthy is fun. Being strong is fun. Having no physical limitations is fun. Getting fit is tough, but being fit is a blast. Keep your eye on the end result and don't get bogged down with the day-to-day of what it takes to get there.

Most of the programs or products out there have one or more of these elements that they market as the value proposition of their program. Belts that melt away belly fat are called **easy**. Bowflex used to advertise if you do 20 minutes a day you'll get fit **quick**. Zumba is dance, so it must be **fun**. What these programs are trying to sell you is that you need their routine to get results. The fact of the matter is that you just need *A* routine, any routine; you can make up your own routine as long as you're consistent. Stick with a routine and you will see results. I am not trying to knock everything that is out there because there are certainly positive attributes to most of these programs and I incorporate some elements from other programs into my routine. For example, I used to own a Bowflex and got my resistance training exclusively from it although I did a lot more than 20 minutes per day and I supplemented with some dumbbell work and body weight work. Sometimes I will vary my routine and do a CrossFit workout when I am on the road, or take a P90X or Insanity class at my regular gym with my wife. These are great programs and I gain a lot of benefit from them, but it is more effective to have an independent routine with weight training as the basis and supplement with these types of group workouts.

My point of all of this is that you need to have a routine that doesn't rely on being easy, quick, or fun. Your routine should be an independent, goal-oriented routine that is going to help you on a daily basis to work toward your goals. A routine that when all else fails – you are out of town, your gym closes, you can't make your class time, whatever – you can find something productive to do on your own. Once you have your routine defined, and are disciplined in it, I definitely recommend incorporating other forms of workout into your regimen.

Chapter 4

The Basics –
Nutrition & Exercise

So you have a reference point in the book to go back to when starting out, I am going to discuss in this chapter exactly what you need to know and do when starting out in a gym or with a nutrition plan. If you are already comfortable with each of these topics, you can move on to the next chapter. I will cover both of these topics in much greater detail in the next two chapters. But if you want a refresher, this chapter will give you a good starting point. For the purposes of this section we are going to put more advanced goals aside for a moment and strictly address the workout and nutrition plan with the overall goal of becoming fit.

Workout Plan - Beginners

First off, my approach is all about weight training. This also goes for women (I will go into this further in the next chapter). Men and women will get much more bang for their buck by investing time in weight training versus strictly cardio exercise. This is a mistake a lot of beginners make when they want to lose weight. They hit the treadmill and hit it hard. In addition, they cut way back on eating, which is a big mistake. You will lose weight right out of the gate, but that will taper off quickly and you will begin to lose muscle mass as well, soon ending up with the dreaded "skinny-fat" look. We want to lose weight *and* gain or tone muscle to get the fitness level and look that we want.

The Plan

As I always say, the most important part of your plan is to actually have a plan. Your plan can't be just to go to the gym. That is way too vague and will leave you wandering around looking for things to do while you are there. What *will* end up happening is instead of getting a good focused workout you will accomplish nothing.

So the first thing you need to do is develop a plan around weight training. Here are some steps in developing your workout plan and getting started in the gym:

1) **Decide on your routine split.** You need to split up the muscles you work on. You don't want to work the same muscles every day as they need rest. Think of how many days per week you are going to work out and what types of exercises you are going to do on those days. There are many variations that I will touch on later, but for the beginner I suggest starting out with a push/pull/legs split. That way you do *pushing* muscles (chest, shoulders, and triceps) one day, then *pulling* muscles (back and biceps) the next day, do your legs the third day, and rest on the fourth day.

2) **Stretch.** I do a lot of stretching, both before and after I exercise. There are a lot of great benefits from stretching. My stretching is focused on mobility and gaining range of motion in my joints, especially in my shoulders and back. This has helped tremendously in my workouts and in alleviating the pain I feel in my joints as I age. For example, through a very specific stretching regimen put together by my physical therapist, I was able to completely eliminate some lower

23

back pain that had been bothering me for months. I would also suggest incorporating some Yoga into your routine, if it is available to you.

3) **Get started in the gym.** In your first week at the gym there is going to be a lot of learning going on. I suggest selecting just a couple of exercises for each muscle to start from the list in Chapter 5 or on www.bodybuilding .com. Once you have the exercises selected you need to see how strong you are. The first few days you should focus on just getting around the gym, familiarizing yourself with the equipment, doing the exercises you chose, and testing different weights until you find a weight that you can barely do for 10 reps. You can then adjust your weight rep range easily. If you want to do 12-15 reps just use a little less weight or if you only want to do six-eight reps, simply up the weight or slow your tempo. This will give you a good starting point and you should do this with each muscle/exercise. You will get a much better feel for a comfortable weight as you progress. If you are a true beginner, it is going to take

you a few weeks to get used to lifting weights (especially free weights). You are going to feel weak, unstable, and you are going to be sore! But trust me you will get more stable and accustomed to the feeling as you progress.

4) **Focus on form.** As you begin lifting make sure you are focused on good form. This will help you prevent injury and build muscle. As you are selecting your weights make sure you are selecting a weight that you can do for the prescribed repetitions while keeping your form throughout.

5) **Don't let weightlifting intimidate you.** There are so many benefits to lifting weights that you should not let it intimidate you into not doing it. Anyone can get in the gym and lift weights. Don't get wrapped up in how much you can lift......check your ego at the door! Focus on your form and your progress and you will be fine. The weight increase will come as you gain experience and build muscle.

6) **Stick to your routine.** It's important to stick with your plan, focus on continuous improvement, and be patient.

7) **Incorporate cardio work into your routine.** Do cardio either at the beginning of your workout or at the end. For weight loss, I recommend doing the cardio at the beginning of your workout. Whether you are starting your workout or finishing it, do your cardio so that it is high intensity but for a short duration (think of it like running wind-sprints instead of a marathon). You can really vary the cardio work by running, biking, or using a treadmill, stair climber, elliptical, or doing a Metcon workout.

Nutrition Plan – Beginners

For beginners, I will keep the nutrition piece very simple. You do not need to be a master chef nor do you need to be wealthy in order to eat healthy. Here are some simple steps to follow:

1) **Eliminate (or drastically reduce) sugar in your diet** Sugar is extremely bad for you and has no nutritional value. In

addition, sugar is addictive, bad for your teeth, increases your risk of developing diabetes, and has fat promoting effects on the body. Does that really sound like something you should be putting in your body? It is tough eliminate sugar all together because it is in so many foods, but if you focus on eating natural (not processed) foods you can really cut back on your intake of sugar.

2) **Eat lots of lean protein** You should get at minimum 0.5g of protein per pound of body weight. If you want to build muscle up that to 1g or more per pound of body weight. I like to get my protein from chicken, pork, beef, venison, and fish. I do eat some processed meats, like sausage, bacon and certain lunch meats, but I try to limit that as much as possible. I apologize to my vegetarian and vegan readers, but I personally do not have experience in protein sources for those of you on these types of diets.

3) **Eat lots of vegetables** The best are green vegetables, such as broccoli, green beans, kale, spinach, brussel sprouts, lettuce, etc.

4) **Get your carbs** from whole grains (oatmeal, rice) and starchy vegetables (potatoes, sweet potatoes).

5) **Eat plenty of good fats** Incorporating good fats into your diet is essential. I use a lot of coconut oil and supplement with MCT oil. I also use full fat everything – salad dressing, mayo, real butter, etc. I don't gorge on this stuff, but I don't buy the low fat as a substitute either.

6) **Drink lots of water**

As you are preparing your meals keep these few simple principles in mind. Try to eat as natural as possible, eliminating processed foods where you can. Generally, your meals should consist of a protein (meat or fish), vegetable, and a rice or potato (not with every meal). I usually grill my meat, but will also occasionally sauté it in oil or butter. The veggies, potato or rice are always steamed and flavored with a little butter, salt, and pepper. If the veggies are high quality I sometimes will just hit them with a little salt and pepper and skip the butter.

I will get more advanced with both the workout

and nutrition in the next two chapters. This chapter hopefully gives you the very basic principles of my thought process when it comes to working out and nutrition. As you read through the workout and nutrition chapters keep these basic principles in mind.

Chapter 5

Workout Plan

In order to be effective in achieving your fitness goals you need to have a workout plan. And as we discussed, the most important element of a workout plan, more important than the plan itself, is simply having a plan and sticking to it. Most people go to the gym with no real focus or direction. They chit chat, play on their cell phones, and accomplish nothing other than feeling good about going to the gym and socializing. In order to make progress toward your goals you need to have a workout plan that you can repeat and track through cycles of days, weeks, and months. By having a routine and keeping track of weight, reps, sets, and times, you can work on improving these elements from workout to workout, or week to week. This will make your progress measureable and allow you to make adjustments as necessary throughout the cycle of your workouts.

The plan you design or choose is going to depend on what you want to achieve, so it is important to first clearly define your goals, as we discussed in previous chapters. For example, you may want to run a marathon in under four hours. In order to achieve that, you are going to need to focus on running so you are going to spend more time on various running activities while still doing some moderate weight training. Also, your weight training will probably look different, meaning more emphasis on lower weights and higher reps. A completely different goal may be to gain 20 lbs of lean muscle mass. In order to achieve that, you will need to go heavy on the weight training and a lot lighter on the amount of running you will be doing. The weight training will look very different than a person with the four-hour marathon goal. Our muscle gainer will likely be doing a workout starting with moderate weights in a moderate rep range, then varying the workout from heavy weights/low reps to low weight/high reps in order to vary the stimulus on the muscles and promote new growth. But remember, no matter the short term goal your long term goal is overall fitness, so don't get overly focused on a singular goal.

The most important point you should take from the previous paragraph is that no matter your ultimate goal, you need to keep the elements of your workout plan diverse and well rounded.

Our runner needs to weight train and our weight trainer needs to have cardio work as a core element of the workout plan. Having a well-rounded workout plan will support your ultimate goal.

Independent Training vs. Group Training

Another important point that I touched on in the introduction is that your workout plan should be based on independent training. I cannot stress enough how important I think this is for building a sustainable strategy. I don't want to discourage anyone from doing group fitness like CrossFit, PiYo, Yoga, Orange Theory, partner workouts, and so forth. I have done most of these classes and they are great! The problem I have is that when your workout revolves around doing it with other people, it allows outside factors (other people) to potentially impact your results. What happens if you are relying on a specific class or workout buddy to provide you with your workout and that instructor leaves or your gym discontinues that class, or you are traveling and there are no classes in the area? How will you get your workout? Most people will simply neglect their workout if that driving force of the group or partner isn't there to support them. Also, it is likely you are getting your motivation to work out from the classes or partner rather than relying on the *discipline* of an independent routine, so when there is no class you have no motivation to workout. I suggest, at least in the beginning, that you develop a solid independent routine for your workout. Once you know you can rely on just yourself to work out, and get results, then I think it is great to complement that with classwork for the competition and camaraderie. I will hit up CrossFit gyms across the country when I am traveling and I meet some great people and get an incredible workout, so I am by no means knocking the effectiveness. CrossFit workouts, in particular, are amazing workouts. I also like to hit up some Yoga classes when I travel. I simply think to have a sustainable routine the base has to be independent workouts. I have seen turnover in gym instructors, I have seen gyms open and close in record time, I have traveled to areas where there is no access to classes; none of which you can control. I like to be in *total* control of my results and you should too.

Let's talk about the structure of your workout plan. Your plan should be designed to give you a minimum five days of workouts per week, but no more than six. You need rest days to combat burnout and allow for adequate muscle recovery. The workouts should also alternate muscle groups or levels of intensity so that you are not working the same muscles day after day. If your workout is heavy on running, swimming, or some other cardio activity, I suggest alternating levels of intensity from day-to-day. For example, one day you might do a series of sprints, the next day a medium distance run, followed by a long distance run on the third day, and so on.

Rest days are extremely important to build into your workout plan. Rest days provide a couple of benefits. One, they allow your muscles to recover, which is when they grow and you see your gains. Two, planned rest days help to combat burnout and the feeling of failure when skipping a workout. I usually do some type of workout all 7 days, but I use one or two days each week as an active recovery day. An active recovery (rest) day is where I will do a very light workout. It is not near as strenuous as a regular workout so it still allows your muscles to recover while also keeping you active. If for some reason I can't get a workout in on that active recovery day I will just take the day off as it is a scheduled rest day.

If you are working out on a four-day cycle – three days on and one day off--you are more likely to suck it up and do a workout on day two of that cycle, particularly if you know you have a planned day off in a couple of days. Building in rest days also gives you the flexibility to adjust. As I am writing this, we are planning an overnight trip to a local ski resort this weekend and I know that I will not get to work out on Saturday. My normal three on/one off work-rest split has my rest day as Friday this week so I simply move into the next scheduled workout on Friday, then use Saturday as my rest day (using skiing as my active recovery activity), then finish up the last two days of my three-day work cycle on Sunday and Monday. By doing this you also end up not feeling bad about not working out on a planned rest day, whereas if you say you are going to work out every day then any missed workout is a missed workout both in your mind and in your plan. If you fail to adhere to your plan, it will feel like a failure. I hate failure and want to avoid it AT ALL COSTS, plan your rest days, and reap the benefits of building in those days in your workout plan.

Deciding on your workout plan (exercises you'll do and amount of weight you'll use) is going to be a lot of trial and error in the beginning. We will discuss what weights/reps you are going to need to figure out and how much weight to use, because you want to use as much weight as you can while doing the required reps. I suggest using a notebook or planner or cell phone notes for your workouts so that you can take it to the gym and track your workouts as you do them. This will allow you to reference previous workouts on the same muscle groups so you can recall the exercises you did along with the weight and reps. As you get more experienced and you have multiple routines down, you may be able to get away without the notes, but I think this is very important in the beginning. I have been doing this for a long time and when I switch my cycles I have a hard time keeping track and still need to maintain notes to this day.

Before we get into specifics there are a couple of things to know:

1) **Decide how much time you want to spend in the gym**. I recommend at least an hour for each workout. That gives you enough time to get in an adequate amount of weight training (approximately 45 minutes) and 15 minutes of intense cardio.

2) **Set limits.** You are going to need to spend the first several days figuring out your limits on the weight you need to use.

3) **Exercise examples.** I list exercises in my plans below. You should also check out www.bodybuilding .com. They have really good video tutorials for almost all of the exercises that I list below. Plus, they have an extensive library of additional exercises by body part, which you can use to build your own plan.

4) **Sets/Reps/# of exercises.** I am going to give you three workout examples, but feel free to adjust the number of exercises you do as well as reps and sets, especially in the beginning while you are building up. I generally do four to five exercises per body part, but you may only have time for three, which is fine.

5) **Make sure weight training is the majority of your workout**. I cannot stress this enough. People, especially people who want to lose weight, get lured into thinking they need to do cardio, cardio, and more cardio in order to get fit.

Your benefits from weight training will far outweigh the benefits from cardio, so no matter your goal *do some weight training.*

Now let's discuss some examples of specific plans you can use. The few options that I am going to share with you are fairly traditional in their approach. Weightlifting and fitness has evolved over time just like everything else. While I mix in new exercise styles into my routine I have my roots in the more traditional lifting and it has served me well. There will be people who read this and criticize my approach because of the movement of CrossFit type workouts, but it has worked for me. And again, my goal in writing this is not to show you how to become an elite bodybuilder or fittest man/woman on the planet, but to give you the knowledge to improve your fitness level and enjoy a healthier life.

I will share the workout plan I have been doing the last few years, and then we will look at it on an annualized basis. When I am looking at an entire year, I like to break it into thirds. I will work out with moderate to heavy weights with moderate to low reps for three months, then drop down and do light weights and high reps for one month. My goals are to increase muscle mass and decrease body fat. The research is inconclusive on what exactly is the best weight/rep range, so this is why I vary it.

Within those workouts I work on a four-day cycle when I am doing the heavier weights. I group muscles and work out for three days then take one day off. I do a push/pull/legs split during this cycle where I work all push muscles in one day (chest, shoulders, triceps), pull muscles (back, biceps) on the second day, and legs on the third day. This allows you to work out day after day because you are working opposing muscles; therefore, you are not wearing them out every day. When I am doing the high rep work, I break my workouts by individual muscle group working one muscle group each day (chest, shoulders, back, arms, legs) so I work out on a five-day cycle with one day off.

In this first three-month cycle, where I am doing moderate to heavy weights, you will see in my example that I give a pretty broad rep range. In this cycle, I generally do not go over 12 reps (unless I am doing a body weight exercise). I give this large rep range in order to keep it flexible. Some weeks I may do three sets of eight reps, other weeks I may do 12 - 10 - eight reps in my three sets, increasing the weight with each set. While other weeks I will do three sets of either

10 or 12 reps. I like to vary this throughout the cycle as it has shown me the best results. I will sometimes do really heavy weights and drop down to only three to five reps per set.

A quick note about the numbers below and what they mean; 3 x 8-12 means 3 sets x 8-12 repetitions per set. So if you are doing an exercise like bench press for 3 x 8-12 you will start by executing it 8-12 times then rest for a period and repeat the exercise 2 more times for 8-12 reps.

So let's start fresh with January and I will map out a workout plan over the course of a year:

January-March – Moderate/heavy weights with moderate to low reps

Day 1 – Chest, shoulders, triceps

Bench press	3 x 8-12
Incline dumbbell press	3 x 8-12
Incline fly	3 x 8-12
Cable cross over	3 x 10-15
Overhead dumbbell press	3 x 8-12
One arm dumbbell press	3 x 8-12
Front and lateral raise combo	3 x 8-12
Upright row	3 x 8-12

Triceps pressdown	3 x 8-12
Dumbbell kickbacks	3 x 8-12
Dips (unweighted)	3 x 25
(weighted)	3 x 10-12
Rope pressdown	3 x 8-12
(finish with drop set)	

Day 2 – Back & Biceps

Pull-ups	3 x failure
Chin ups	3 x failure
Bent over row (or machine row)	3 x 8-12
One arm row	3 x 8-12
Hammer curl	3 x 8-12
Dumbbell curl	3 x 8-12
Preacher curl	3 x 8-12
Reverse curl	3 x 8-12

Day 3 – Legs

Squat	3 x 8-12
Power Clean or Snatch	3 x 8-12
Deadlift	3 x 8-12
Barbell hip thrust	3 x 8-12
Walking lunges	3 x 8-12
Calf raises	3 x 75-100

*changing angles of feet (in, neutral, out)

Day 4 – Rest

Start cycle over

Here are a few key points when using this route:

1) **Weight/Reps.** This weight/rep range is best for building muscle (gaining size) and gaining strength.

2) **Order of Exercises.** Each day work your body parts in order from largest to smallest on that given day. As you can see from what I have listed, when I am on a Chest/Shoulders/Triceps day I do my chest first, then shoulders, then finish up with triceps. The reason for this is that as you are working the larger muscles, each smaller muscle is engaged in that exercise so you should just progress right down through to the smallest muscle. This will optimize your training and allow you to get the most out of your workout. I have the exercises listed in the order they should be done.

3) **Rest.** Allow only 60-90 seconds of rest between sets in this heavy cycle. If you do

four exercises for each muscle group with no more than 60-90 seconds of rest between sets you can do all of these workouts in one hour.

4) **Length of workout.** If you have longer to workout, simply add additional sets or additional exercises to each muscle group. I use four exercises each as a minimum for me. If I have more time I will go up to six exercises for each muscle group. Conversely, if you are just beginning and/or don't have the time, drop down to three exercises for each. I would not recommend going less than that because you want the weight training to be the bulk of your workout.

Cardio

During this cycle I do cardio after every workout. I alternate between using the stairclimber, rowing machine, running, biking or, as I mentioned earlier, I sometimes substitute activities such as Jiu-Jitsu, hockey, CrossFit/exercise class, or hiking/hunting for cardio. I admit I hate every minute of my cardio work, but I do it anyway as it is a crucial part of my fitness routine. So when it comes to cardio I like to do very intense exercise for shorter durations of time. I typically go as hard as I can for as little as 10 minutes to as long as 20 minutes. The intensity of cardio all depends on the intensity of my weight lifting and other activities I may have planned for that day. This has been effective for me and allows me to keep my total workout time to 60-90 minutes.

Metabolic Conditioning

Recently, I have been doing Metabolic Conditioning (Metcon) workouts at the end of my weight training instead of cardio. A Metcon workout uses a combination of high intensity resistance movements followed by short rest periods for successive rounds. It is high intensity and generally short duration (8-20 minutes). I have found this to be the most effective method of burning fat for me. You can pull Metcon workouts from any CrossFit gym website. I simply go onto a website of a CrossFit gym that I have visited and look at their daily WOD (Workout of the Day) and I will do just that element for my cardio.

As I have indicated from the onset of this book, my methods are rooted in traditional resistance training, but I have been open to adapting. In recent years, with the explosion in popularity of CrossFit, which incorporates a lot of Metcon workouts, you have seen weight and fitness training methods really change. That said, CrossFit and Metcon workouts still have elements of traditional lifting movements in them. So, I strongly recommend that you incorporate some Metcon workouts into your routine as a complement to your lifting. This way you will reap the benefits of both types of exercise.

Here is a quick example of what a Metcon workout would look like:

7 Rounds for Time:

10 Wallballs (20 lb ball for men/14 lb ball for women)

10 Pull-ups (if you can't do the pull-ups do jumping pull-ups)

*9 minute time cap

If you are wondering a wallball is where you stand in front of a wall with a medicine ball, squat down then throw it up to a 10-foot target. You then catch the ball on the way down and repeat.

So in this workout above you have to complete 7 rounds without stopping in under 9 minutes. As you can see, doing 10 reps of each exercise with no rest will be incredibly tasking on your muscles, heart, and lungs.

Abs/Traps

I also do abs and traps/neck every day. When I am doing abs I choose four exercises and do three sets. I vary my ab exercises every day and focus on exercises that not only work the abs, but work my core muscles. You get far more benefit from core work than you do just working the superficial ab muscles. For my traps, I do shrugs, some lying neck work, and a neck harness. When I am doing the shrugs and neck harness I do three sets of each. I incorporate these into my workout while I am resting between sets for other exercises so it doesn't add time to my workout. For example, if I am benching, once I finish a set I will hop up and do shrugs during my 60 seconds of rest. I overwork these muscles because I think they can take it and I think a thick neck/traps and tight abs just look damn good!

This is my basic routine for this three-month period. I will vary this a bit alternating in different exercises, weight/rep ranges, and intensity. I list the exercises in this workout as an example for a given week, but I have a list of eight to 12 exercises for each muscle group that I select from. At the end of this chapter I will include a list of exercises that I use.

For month number four in the cycle I will follow the routine described below:

April – Low Weights and High Reps

Day 1 – Chest

Bench press	3 x 20-25
Dumbbell incline press	3 x 20-25
Incline fly	3 x 20-25
Machine press	3 x 20-25
Cable cross over	3 x 20-25

Day 2 – Back

Pull-ups	3 x failure
Chin ups or ring pullups	3 x failure

Cable pulldowns	3 x 20-25
Machine row	3 x 20-25
Bent over row	3 x 20-25

Day 3 – Shoulders

Overhead dumbbell press	3 x 20-25
Push press	3 x 20-25
Front raise	3 x 20-25
Lateral raise	3 x 20-25
Upright row	3 x 20-25

Day 4 – Legs

Squat	3 x 20-25
Power Clean or Snatch	3 x 20-25
Deadlift	3 x 20-25
Barbell hip thrust	3 x 20-25
Walking lunges	3 x 20-25
Calf raises	3 x 75

*changing angles of feet (in, neutral, out)

Day 5 – Biceps & Triceps*

Triceps pressdown	3 x 20-25
Dumbbell kickbacks	3 x 20-25
Skull crusher	3 x 20-25
Dips (unweighted)	3 x 25

Rope pressdown	3 x 20-25
(finish with drop set)	

Hammer curl	3 x 20-25
Dumbbell curl	3 x 20-25
Preacher curl	3 x 20-25
Reverse curl	3 x 20-25
Rope curl	3 x 20-25
(finish with drop set)	

Day 6 – Rest

Day 7– Light total body workout and light cardio

*An important thing to note about my arm day in this cycle is that I superset every arm exercise, which means I match up a bicep exercise with a triceps exercise and do them back-to-back with no rest. They are opposing muscles so when one is working the other is not, which is why you can do this. I feel this adds to the level of intensity and helps get you through the workout more efficiently. I also finish each arm routine with a drop set. This is where I do the exercise, but on the third set once I do the reps to failure I lower the weight and keep doing sets to failure until I get to where I am doing them with no weight.

I have found this routine to be good for

maintaining muscle mass and leaning up because of the high intensity weight training. I do a minimum of five exercises per muscle group during this routine and as many as seven. I only rest 30 seconds in between sets during this routine. The minimal rest with the high reps leads to a really intense workout. So, in this cycle, I reduce my amount of cardio because of the intensity and cardio vascular effect of the weight lifting. Again, you can do these workouts in 60 minutes or less. If you want to go longer just add additional exercises.

Cardio

During this cycle I do cardio every other day. Because of the intensity of this weight lifting routine I do not feel that I need cardio every day. I still alternate between a stairclimber, rowing machine, running, biking, or as I mentioned earlier I sometimes substitute activities such as Jiu-Jitsu, hockey, CrossFit/exercise class, or hiking/hunting for cardio. I subscribe to the same short duration high intensity work as I always do with my cardio work.

I will also sub in a short Metcon workout in lieu of doing cardio during this cycle as well. I have really come to prefer the Metcon workouts instead of strictly cardio as I feel you can really push yourself in those short durations and see some great gains.

I still do abs and traps/neck every day. When I am doing abs I choose four exercises and do three sets. When I am doing the shrugs and neck harness I do three sets of each.

This is my basic routine for this one-month period. When I finish with this I will start over with the same routine that I started in January and run that routine for three months (May-July) then do this routine again in August. So it's a four-month cycle that I repeat three times per year.

Full Body Workout

As an alternative to these split workouts you can also do a full body workout. I do not often go the full body route, but it can be effective. If I do a period of a full body routine I will only do two to three exercises per body part and I will work out every other day, repeating this routine. In this workout, to keep it intense rest only 30 seconds between sets. You can also superset working opposing muscles with no rest. For example, if you are working a pull muscle like biceps, instead of resting you can go straight to a push muscle like triceps and do a set of those instead of resting. You can do the same thing with back (pull muscle) and chest (push muscle). This increases the intensity of the workout and lessens the duration.

Here is an example of a full body routine:

Day 1

Chest

Bench press	3 x 10-12
Dumbbell incline press	3 x 10-12

Back

Pull-ups	3 x failure
Machine row	3 x 10-12

Shoulders

Overhead dumbbell press	3 x 10-12
Front raise	3 x 10-12
Lateral raise	3 x 10-12

Legs

| Squat | 3 x 10-12 |
| Deadlift | 3 x 10-12 |

Triceps

Triceps pressdown	3 x 10-12
Rope pressdown	3 x 10-12
(finish with drop set)	

Biceps

Hammer curl	3 x 10-12
Dumbbell curl	3 x 10-12
(finish with drop set)	

This routine works well if you are truly tight on time and can't be in the gym every day. This routine does have some good benefits in that you are breaking down all of your muscles at once and you reap metabolic benefits for days after your workout.

During this cycle I do cardio after every workout and on the days in between I do a Metcon workout. For the cardio, I alternate between stairclimber, rowing machine, running, biking or sometimes I will substitute activities such as Jiu-Jitsu, hockey, or hiking/hunting. Once again, I hate every minute of my cardio work, but I do it anyway as it is a crucial part of my fitness routine. I typically go as hard as I can for as little as 10 minutes to as long as 20 minutes.

I still do abs and traps/neck every day. When I am doing abs I choose four exercises and do three sets. When I am doing the shrugs and neck harness I do three sets of each.

Here are a couple of important points to note regardless of the cycle in the routine:

1) **Stretching.** I stretch before and after every workout, and I stretch on my off days. I sometimes stretch multiple times per day. I feel that stretching is extremely important. It not only helps with the flexibility in your muscles, but also the mobility in your joints. Having flexibility and mobility will allow you to do more diverse exercises and movements in the gym. I will occasionally do a Yoga class in my travels. If you can incorporate Yoga into your routine, I would highly recommend it.

2) **Adjust your weight accordingly**. If you are doing a workout where you are doing three sets of eight reps, adjust the weight so you can barely do that set/rep range. You don't want to use a weight that you could easily lift 15 times, but only do it eight times. You always want to be flirting with failure while maintaining good form....this is where progress is made.

3) **Focus on continuous progress**. Keep track of the weight and reps you are doing and try to improve on your lift every couple of weeks. You don't want to be benching 200 lbs for three sets of eight week after week for months. You will not see any progress. When an exercise starts becoming easy to do at a given weight, add more weight.

4) **BE INTENSE**. Manage the intensity of your workout. I see many people in the gym who just go through the motions. Get in there and workout with a purpose! If you are in the gym for 60 minutes that's 4.2% of your entire day. It is such a small period of time so use it wisely. Commit to going hard in that short amount of time.

5) **Don't eat prior to your workout.** For the best results in burning fat you should workout in the morning and do so before eating. This will allow your body to fuel itself from stored fat, thus burning it rather than the quick access to the fuel you put in by eating before your workout. If mornings aren't your thing and you like to work out in the afternoon or evening, then try to fast for a couple of hours prior to your workout in order to get a similar benefit. For the absolute best result, if you have the time to do it, do your cardio in the morning after a long overnight fast and do your weight training later in the day when you can eat before and after your workout. This gives you the benefits of burning fat coming off a fasting period and being able to fuel your weight training in a separate session in the afternoon or evening.

6) **Eat right after your workout.** Your muscles need protein as soon as possible following your workout. Try to get some protein rich food or a protein supplement into your body within an hour of your

workout. By not eating before and eating right after you can have the benefits of burning fat and building muscle at the same time.

Here are sample exercises for each muscle group to use for the workouts I have mentioned:

Chest – Bench press, incline bench, decline bench, dumbbell press, dumbbell incline press, dumbbell fly, dumbbell incline fly, peck deck, cable crossover, pullovers, ring push-up, medicine ball push-up.

Shoulders – Military press, dumbbell press, one arm dumbbell press (standing), push press, upright row, front raise, lateral raise, handstand pushups.

Triceps – Kickbacks, dip (bars), dip (bench), dip (rings), pressdown, reverse grip pressdown, rope pressdown, one arm overhead extension, skull crushers.

Back – Pull-ups, chin-ups, rope climb, cable pull downs, cable rows, bent-over rows, one-arm rows, machine pull downs.

Biceps – Hammer curl, standing dumbbell curl, seated incline dumbbell curl, concentration curl, preacher curl, reverse curl, cable curl, cable rope curl.

Legs – Squat, front squat, deadlift, straight leg deadlift, barbell hip thrust, leg press, hack squat, walking lunge, weighted barbell step up, calf machine.

Abs/Core – Decline weighted crunches, crunches, hollow rockers, arched rocker, hollow rocker to tuck, L-Sit, L-Sit pull-up, L-sit toes to bar, toes to bar, barbell rollout, bottoms up, barbell climb, push-up walkouts, fallouts (rings).

Traps/Neck – Shrugs, neck harness

Again, check out www.bodybuilding.com for some different ideas on exercises and for video tutorials of all of the exercises listed above. This site has an excellent library of exercises. Don't feel like you have to use the exercises listed. Each exercise has its pros and cons so just pick some exercises and go with them. I like to vary my exercises with every workout so no two workouts look the same. I may have an exercise or two for each muscle group that I do every workout, but I change the majority of the exercises I use every single workout. The benefit of varying your workout is hitting muscles from different angles all the time.

These routines are just some examples of things I have done. They have served me quite well over the last few years and will, hopefully, do the same for you. As you can see, there is nothing here that you probably haven't seen before, but it is simply spelled out and organized. I am constantly exploring new methods and routines and I would encourage you to do the same. As I write this I am researching some kettlebell work and plan on incorporating some of those exercises into my routine. So feel free to explore different exercises and mix up your routine. What you should take from this chapter is that you need to have some structure in the form of a routine. Use mine or make your own, it doesn't matter as long as you have one and make sure you are working out with a level of intensity that is pushing your limits. As long as you are sticking to the set/rep/# of exercises in your routine you will be good to go.

Free weights vs. Machines

Given the choice between free weights and machines I will choose free weights every time. Machines are fine to use, but free weights are the preferred method. When using machines, you are isolating muscles, whereas free weights and compound movement exercises activate more muscles than just those you are working directly. You will see much greater gains from free weights than you will machines. Free weights take some getting used to because until you develop those stabilizing muscles many of the exercises will feel awkward and you will feel weak, but as you develop your muscles you will see that you will gain strength quickly. All that said, you can certainly substitute machine exercises as well. If you are a beginner, don't have a spotter, or are short on time machines can be a great alternative to free weights. The types of machines will vary greatly depending on the gym and the brand of machines, but they are generally self-explanatory and easy to use with illustrations on them.

Importance of Weight Training

Regardless of your goals – weight loss or muscle gain – weight or resistance training needs to be the foundation of your workout plan. The benefits you gain from weight training are not only building muscle, but also fat loss. When you weight train you are actually damaging your muscles and the recovery from that damage is what builds them up. But what you also get from this is that your body is expending energy to repair your muscles for days after your workout, so you get the added benefit of the weight training for days versus the immediate effect of the cardio work. I have found it to be much more effective to utilize weight training in weight loss than strictly cardio. If you are just going to the gym and hammering the treadmill for 60 minutes or doing an aerobics class for 60 minutes you will see results, but they won't be as dramatic or lasting as if you were weight training. In addition, by only doing cardio any weight loss you experience will leave you looking soft or "skinny-fat," which most people don't want. Use weight training as the basis of your fitness plan and you will build muscle and tone up while losing weight which will lead to a much better look. As a general rule, if you are looking to lose weight I would go with the high rep/low weight/high intensity weight training along with the short high intensity cardio. If you are looking to gain muscle/strength, then go with the low rep/high weight workout.

Women & Weight Training

I want to touch quickly on women and weight training. Women need to weight train! I hear from countless women that they don't want to weight train because they don't want to bulk up. In fact, I personally know many women who do nothing but exercise classes and/or cardio work. This is a total myth. Women simply do not produce enough testosterone to bulk up from doing some basic (or even moderate) weight training. If you do the proper weight training and pair it with proper nutrition you do not need to worry about bulking up. You simply need to control the food you are putting into your body. The weights are merely going to sculpt your muscles. The growth will come when you couple that sculpting with fuel (food) and supplements. As a woman you should be weight training and monitoring your food to stay healthy and toned without being overly muscular. If you don't believe in this approach, go onto Instagram. I search a lot of fitness information there and if you have ever done the same you know there are a myriad of fitness models posting photos and videos of their workouts. If you take notice, these women are some of the best built women you will ever see and you rarely see them post a video of themselves doing cardio work. They almost always post videos of themselves doing some kind of weight or resistance training. This is not a coincidence. These women are proof that weight training works for women as well.

Whatever your routine, you should try to adhere to it as strictly as possible. I travel for work often so I cannot always do my workouts exactly as I would like. I sometimes have to modify them for a hotel gym that has minimal equipment. I sometimes have to do a body weight workout when no gym is available. Or I will sometimes take a CrossFit class that doesn't necessarily line up with my workout plan that day, but that is the best thing available. The most important thing is that you do something. Your workout plan will map out the days you should be working out and the days you should be resting. On the workout days, even if you can't make it to your regular gym or don't have access to the equipment you need, it is a day designated for a workout so do something, which is always better than nothing. No matter where you are or what equipment you have, you will always have your body and there is plenty you can do with just that even though you may not like it.

Remember workout days are workout days and rest days are rest days. Chances are that a day will come when you won't feel great on a workout day, but workout anyway. You may not feel great on a rest day, then go ahead and rest. There are going to be days when you just plain don't feel like working out, but you need to do it anyway. That's the differentiator. Everyone can workout when they feel like it. Continuous and sustainable progress is made by putting in the work even when you don't want to do it. Getting out of your routine by missing your workout, ending up over weight, and out of shape, starts with the first missed workout, so NEVER miss one. Remember the more you accept small failures, like one missed workout in your plan, the easier it will become to accept bigger and bigger failures. You will go from missing a workout one day to missing a whole week to not working out at all. If you NEVER miss, you will NEVER be at risk of spiraling out of control and breaking your routine.

Chapter 6

Nutrition

Before we begin, as with any change in diet or exercise, it is important to consider the impact on your body and consult a physician before making a drastic change.

Your eating habits are a key component to your overall fitness plan. In my opinion, a good nutrition plan is much more important than a good workout routine. You can absolutely kill the results of your workout routine with a poor diet. I see guys at the gym who are big and strong, but have big midsections and couldn't get out of their own way. If your goal is only strength or size and not overall fitness, you can get away with pretty poor eating habits and still get strong. However, if you really want to be fit and feel great, then you need to put some thought and commitment into what you eat.

If you had to choose between eating right and working out, eating right will get you results on its own. Food is your fuel, so if you are working out and not fueling your body with the right foods, as a complement to your workout, then you are not going to see the results that you want.

Adhering to a strict diet is difficult because bad food is generally made for convenience; it's cheaper, instantly gratifying, and usually very tasty. It is always in front of us. Whether you are at home or on the road, think about all of the things that are quick and easy to grab and eat when you are hungry; chips, pretzels, candy bars, candy, cookies.....the list is endless and absolutely terrible for you.

I like to practice a fairly strict nutrition plan, but not go crazy. I think if you don't indulge a little bit that it makes you prone to cheating and also is just no fun. There are several schools of thought here. You can practice an ultra-strict diet six days a week and have an all-out cheat day each week. I have never gone that route, but I have read enough to know that it can be effective. I take a little different approach. I may "cheat" on any given day, but my cheating is not a binge. In fact, I don't like to think of it as cheating......I live! Living sometimes involves eating some things you like, but I do so in moderation. I love to eat so I think you will find my nutrition plan very sustainable. I try to eat very clean 90% of the time and leave room to indulge every so often when I see fit. By doing this I am very concentrated on making sure I am eating healthy 90% of the time so when I am on the road at a nice restaurant and I finish a "clean" meal, like a steak with fresh steamed vegetables. I then have no problem finishing it off with a Crème Brule for dessert. That said, with every bite I take I am thinking about what I am going to need to do the next morning to work it off. If you have the mentality of thinking about every meal you eat, and its consequences on your body, you will find it much easier to stick to your plan

If you noticed, I don't use the word diet much. I think that the word diet has a negative connotation in the minds of most people, signifying something that is a burden and only temporary. The word diet puts me off as soon as I hear it. I tend to use the term nutrition plan or eating plan instead of diet. But whatever you want to call it, just think of it as a healthy, sustainable way to eat rather than something you are suffering through. A nutrition plan is not a diet in the traditional sense, where all you hear is "don't eat this" and "don't eat that." My plan is very simple – eat foods that have high protein, good carbs, and high fat (but good fat). It doesn't matter what you eat or when you eat it, just make sure to maximize your protein, minimize your carbs and minimize your bad fats. There will be room in there to eat anything you like within moderation. You can get away with that as long as you put some thought into your meals and try to stick to some very basic principles.

What I have done is conditioned myself to enjoy eating foods that are much better and more satisfying for my body. If you get your satisfaction from sweets and potato chips know that it will gratify your taste buds, but not your body. Change those snacks to beef jerky, yogurt, nuts, or berries and your body will thank you. In fact, your body will start craving those foods, which will in turn fuel it. You want to intake foods that are not only delicious to eat, but also have a great impact on your body. The key is not to stop eating, but to actually eat more often, eat smaller portions, and make sure you eat the right things.

Protein

I can bet that almost everyone reading this book needs to increase their protein intake. Protein is the key component in packing on muscle. Building muscle leads to burning fat, which helps our overall fitness. As a general rule of thumb I think the average person should take in about 0.5g-1g of protein per pound of body weight. So if you weigh 200 lbs you would be eating at least 100g of protein per day. I like to try to take in 1g per pound. So at 200 lbs I try to take in 200g of protein. This helps with my heavy workout routine and the muscle building process. If you fall anywhere in the 0.5-1g per pound you should be fine.

For women, I would suggest sticking with that 0.5g per pound, especially if you are looking to lose weight and you don't want to gain a lot of muscle mass. You still need to get an adequate amount of protein because even if your goal is to lose weight you should still be doing resistance training and looking to tone muscle, and you are going to need to intake protein to achieve that.

You should get as much protein as you can from natural sources, such as meats, eggs, milk, nuts, etc. I supplement a little to get 200g per day, but I try to keep that to a minimum. If you have ever tried, it is really hard to eat that much protein naturally. Supplementation is great, but if you can get your required amount from natural sources go that route first. I think you should vary the sources from where you get your protein. I eat chicken, beef, pork, seafood (all kinds), cottage cheese, eggs, milk, almonds, and

Greek yogurt. Chicken is probably the staple in my protein diet. I am also heavy on the red meat – usually beef, but also venison certain times of year. I eat three to four steaks each week. Red meat gets bashed a lot in the press as being unhealthy, but the more I have eaten it the better results I have seen in getting lean and building muscle from eating red meat, especially venison. Research has also shown that the effects from red meat are not nearly as bad as once thought. Saturated fats in junk food have a far worse impact on your health than the fat in red meat.

When looking at sources of protein you need to make sure you don't overlook incorporating seafood in your normal diet. Aside from being high in protein, seafood contains very healthy fats and Omega 3 fatty acids. I not only have seafood as a staple in my plan, but I also supplement it with seafood products. This is an area in my nutrition plan that I need to pay particular attention to. It is hard to make sure you are getting enough seafood, especially if you do not live close to the coast where options are readily available. In rural Western PA, where I live, it can be difficult to find quality seafood. In addition to it being hard to find, fish and other seafood are typically harder to prepare than other proteins. It takes a bit more skill and knowledge in the kitchen to prepare a good piece of fish. So you just need to work a little harder to make sure you are incorporating these foods in your diet.

Carbohydrates

Unlike protein, I would bet most people are eating too many carbs, in particular sugars. When putting together your eating plan, the first thing that everyone should do is **stop eating sugar,** or at the very least drastically cut back on it. Sugar should be an indulgence, not a staple in your plan. Sugar is a simple carbohydrate which adds absolutely zero value to the muscle building process and is converted to fat stores in your body. There is no benefit to eating sugar other than it tastes good. You could completely cut this out of your diet and not see any ill effects. I try to eliminate all sugar from my normal eating. In fact, I all but quit eating fruit; a food that people generally think is healthy, because fruit contains a high level of sugars. I will eat strawberries, blueberries, or blackberries a few times a week because I think it is important to have some fruit in your diet and those fruits provide the most benefit, but other than that I am fruit free. You want to lose weight and cut fat, then cut out the sugar.

Now I am not one of these crazy Atkins people who say eat tons of fat and protein and zero carbs. My idea of a healthy eating plan is somewhere in the middle. I think you should eat plenty of fats and protein, but I also think you should eat your fair share of carbs. That said, it should be the right carbs. If I wasn't clear in the prior paragraph sugars are not the right carbs. I like to get my carbs from oatmeal, rice, potatoes, sweet potatoes, nuts, quinoa, beans, etc. These carbs tend to give you the energy that you need and are a much healthier addition to your meals.

Fats

Fats are a misunderstood component of eating. You go to the grocery store and everyone is marketing low fat this, fat free that. Everyone thinks you need to cut fat and eat fat free to lose weight. Nothing could be further from the truth. I eat full fat everything. I recently started adding straight up fat to my plan through supplementation and I have never seen a more drastic cut in weight/body fat in all the years I have been working out. You just need to be cognizant of the kinds of fats you are introducing into your body. When I say I am adding fat I don't mean I am stuffing my face with corn chips. I am adding good fats, which are unsaturated medium chain triglycerides. I get these from using products like MCT oil or coconut oil. I will add these directly to my coffee or protein shake. These fats are not stored in the body like other fats and sugars, but are actually used by the body as energy, kind of like a substitute for carbs.

There are some fats you want to stay away from and those are the trans fats that you find in processed foods like corn chips and margarine. These are extremely unhealthy for you and are actually being fazed out of the food industry. But there are still products out there that contain these. So, focus on getting your fats from natural sources like coconut oil, MCT oil, meats, eggs, etc.

Calories

This may be a controversial statement, but I absolutely never look at my caloric intake because I am always ok with putting on lean muscle mass. Some people may disagree with this, but it is my philosophy that if you are eating the right foods then you don't need to be worried about calories. You can stuff your face with grilled chicken and steamed broccoli all day! Everyone gets wrapped up in calories. If you take care to monitor the amount of proteins, fats (good fats), and carbs (good, complex carbs) your intake of calories will take care of itself. You will only need to monitor your calories if you really need to drop pounds. In that case, even if you are eating right, while it won't have a negative impact on your body composition you will need to cut back on the amount (of calories). In order to achieve weight loss, you will need to burn more calories than you are consuming.

Sample Eating Plan

In this section I am going to illustrate a one-week sample of my actual meals and snacks. My meals consist of good portions of lean meat, veggies, and sometimes rice, potatoes, or beans. It is a simple plan to stick to.

Day 1

Pre-Workout: Coffee with one to two tablespoons of MCT Oil

Breakfast: Three or four eggs
                 Slice of cheese melted in eggs
                 Half avocado sliced on top of eggs
                 6-8 oz steak

Coffee

Snack: Protein shake

Lunch: Salad
                10-oz chicken
                Mozzarella cheese (grated)
                Caesar Dressing

Snack: Sardines

Snack: Protein bar

Dinner: 12-oz chicken, green beans, sweet
potato

Snack: Cottage Cheese
                *Mix in almonds for a little added
                protein and flavor

Day 2

Pre-Workout: Coffee with one to two tablespoons
of MCT Oil

Breakfast: Three or four eggs
                Four sausage links

¼ cup oatmeal
Coffee

Snack: Protein bar

Lunch: Salad
              10-oz steak
              Mozzarella cheese (grated)
              Caesar Dressing

Snack: Smoked oysters

Snack: Protein shake, almonds

Dinner: 12 oz Salmon, brussel sprouts, rice

Snack: Greek Yogurt
              *I mix in some protein powder
              with the yogurt and top it off with
              a small scoop of cool whip for
              added flavor.....eats like a dessert

Day 3

Pre-Workout: Coffee with one to two tablespoons
of MCT Oil

Breakfast: Three or four eggs

Mozzarella cheese (grated) melted
Half avocado sliced on top of eggs
6-8 oz chicken
Salsa
Coffee

Snack: Protein shake

Lunch: Salad
                10-oz chicken
                Mozzarella cheese (grated)
                Caesar dressing

Snack: Sardines

Snack: Protein bar

Dinner: 12-oz steak, asparagus,
                mushrooms

Snack: Cottage Cheese
                *Mix in almonds for a little added
                protein and flavor

Day 4

Pre-Workout: Coffee with one to two tablespoons
of MCT Oil

Breakfast: Three or four eggs
Four slices of bacon
¼ cup oatmeal
Coffee

Snack: Protein bar

Lunch: Salad
10-oz steak
Mozzarella cheese (grated)
Caesar dressing

Snack: Smoked oysters

Snack: Protein shake, almonds

Dinner: 12-oz Venison steak, chopped
spinach, rice

Snack: Greek Yogurt
*Mix in some protein powder and
top with a small scoop of cool
whip.

Day 5

Pre-Workout: Coffee with one to two tablespoons
of MCT Oil

Breakfast: Three or four eggs
               Slice of cheese melted in eggs
               Half an avocado sliced on top of
               6-8 oz steak
               Coffee

Snack: Protein shake

Lunch: Salad
               10-oz chicken
               Mozzarella cheese (grated)
               Caesar dressing

Snack: Sardines

Snack: Protein bar

Dinner: 12-oz pork chops, broccoli, sweet
potato

Snack: Cottage Cheese
               *Mix in almonds for a little added
               protein and flavor

Day 6

Pre-Workout: Coffee with one to two tablespoons of MCT Oil

Breakfast:	Three or four eggs Four sausage links ¼ cup oatmeal Coffee
Snack:	Protein bar
Lunch:	Salad 10-oz steak Mozzarella cheese (grated) Caesar dressing
Snack:	Smoked oysters
Snack:	Protein shake, almonds
Dinner:	12-oz haddock filet (lightly breaded), green beans
Snack:	Greek Yogurt *Mix in protein powder with your yogurt and top with a small scoop of cool whip.

Day 7

Pre-Workout: Coffee with one or two tablespoons of MCT Oil

Breakfast: Three or four eggs
              Mozzarella cheese (grated) melted
              Half avocado sliced on top of eggs
              6-8 oz chicken
              Salsa
              Coffee

Snack: Protein bar

Lunch: Salad
              Mozzarella cheese (grated)
              Caesar dressing
              10-oz tuna (eaten separately)

Snack: Smoked oysters

Snack: Protein shake, almonds

Dinner: 12-oz steak, asparagus, baked
              potato

Snack: Greek Yogurt
              *Mix in protein powder with your

yogurt and top with a small scoop
of cool whip

In my plan I eat three main meals then snack a lot in between. I try to stick to something high protein, low sugar for my snack. You will also see that every day I eat either sardines or smoked oysters. These aren't the greatest tasting snacks (actually the oysters are pretty good), but if you recall I indicated earlier that I struggle to eat enough seafood, which has a lot of great benefits so I use these items because they are quick and easy to get no matter where you live. If you don't like sardines, it takes about 30 seconds to choke them down so you can get past it! If you can't do that, no big deal. Just sub in another high protein, low carb snack instead.

As you can see, I am primarily a meat and vegetables guy. Usually, if I eat oatmeal with breakfast I will skip the potato for dinner, and if I don't eat oatmeal at breakfast then I will do a potato at dinner. Protein is a given in my diet and takes little thought. Most fats I get are derived from the proteins, the MCT oil, coconut oil, canola oil, or butter that I cook with. The only thing I have to pay attention to each day is my carb intake. Also, I eat either cottage cheese or plain Greek yogurt every single night as my snack, usually between 8:00pm-9:00pm, and that is the last thing I eat until the next morning.

Don't get wrapped up in the exact foods I have included in my sample meal plan. My nutrition plan can be summed up very simply as limit your processed foods and eat plants and animals. If it didn't walk on four legs, have wings, or grow out of the ground, then don't eat it. If anything happened to your food (meat or veggie) other than someone killing or harvesting it, then limit your intake of it. Most of your food should be meat, vegetables, and natural grains or starches. Again, don't be insane with this. Aim to eat this way 90% of the time and leave yourself that 10% of your intake to eat some of those processed foods or desserts, if need be.

The foods I choose to eat are pretty simple to prepare. I have really come to enjoy cooking and will prepare more complex meals on occasion. I think you really need to embrace your time in the kitchen and find a way to enjoy it if you are going to commit to healthy eating habits. That said, start off with simple, quick, easy to prepare meals like I have listed in my plan.

I cook almost all of my meat on the grill and the other foods with butter, canola oil, or coconut oil. With the butter, you really get some added flavor. I don't worry about the added fat with these ingredients because the fats, especially in the coconut oil, can be very good for you. If you find yourself getting hung up on fat content try using coconut oil as your cooking agent when you are baking or cooking meat or veggies on the stove top.

I definitely indulge (or cheat). There are very few things that are absolutely off limits to me in my nutrition plan. Those things are mainly items that are low protein and high sugar like candy (hard candy, lollipops, Skittles, gummy bears) or candy bars. These items add no nutritional value. Outside of that I will occasionally indulge in a broad spectrum of things. For example, I love Chinese food and I get it with my family once a week. While I don't really have a weakness for sweets there are a few things I really enjoy, like crème Brule, cheesecake, chocolate chip cookies, and Chocolate Delight (a pudding dessert my family makes). And in the summer my kids love ice cream, so I will have some ice cream with them every week or every other week. My goal is to be healthy and well built. By no means do I have a perfect body and I could certainly drop more body fat, but I like to enjoy some foods and that is a trade-off I am willing to accept. Again, my whole approach is to develop a fit sustainable body that is well balanced. With my nutrition plan you will see benefits and get fit, but it is not designed to get you down to single digit body fat percentage. It is, however, effective, sustainable, and will lead to a lean, fit body.

Fasting

Fasting can be a great way to get your appetite under control and if done properly can be very healthy for you. Here are some benefits to fasting:

1) Appetite control/eating patterns
2) Weight loss
3) Improved metabolism
4) Improved insulin sensitivity
5) Longevity
6) Improved cognitive function
7) Improved immune system
8) Improved self-awareness/enlightenment
9) Improved complexion

For the purposes of what we are trying to accomplish we are going to focus on the appetite control/eating patterns, weight loss, and improved metabolism.

When I talk about fasting I mean intake nothing but water for your fasting period. I prefer to fast frequently for short periods of time. I do not do long fasting periods very often as I lose weight pretty quickly with my active lifestyle. I suggest starting off with a 12-hour fast. Once you do that, wait about a week and try an 18-hour fast. Work your way up to a 24-hour fast. Once you can do that without any issue, you can move on to attempting multi-day fasts (up to 72 hours). If you do this properly you will find that going long periods of time without eating will have no impact on your daily activities. Once you break the mental barrier of not eating you will see that it is not a factor. On days I fast I do all of my normal activities and workouts without any issues. Just remember that you need to build this up. If you can't do 12 hours try going six to eight hours and building yourself up. Once you get this down you will find it much easier to control urges to eat as well.

I try to fast every day for 10-12 hours. I get up at 4:30am and get to the gym around 5:00am. After I finish my workout and shower it is 6:30am. I usually eat immediately following my workout as I like to fuel that workout quickly, but every few days I will hold off on eating until around 7:30am or 8:00am. The first food I eat starts my timer on eating. I will then try to eat every couple of hours for roughly the next 12 hours. If you can reduce this window to nine to10 hours that is even more optimal, but it can be difficult to do if you have a tight schedule or evening activities that push your meals to later in the evening. If I am not busy with work in the morning, I will try to hold off on eating my first meal until 10:00am or 11:00am. This starts the timing on that window later and allows me to eat further into the evening. I do this because I prefer to eat later in the evening. By doing this you will automatically fast 12-15 hours every day. And yes it counts as fasting if you use your sleeping time to coincide with your fast.

One thing I want to make clear about fasting is that fasting isn't dieting. I am not telling you to eat less. I am simply telling you to eat all the food you plan on eating, but do it in a specified (planned) period of time and build in long intervals where you don't eat anything. Your protein or caloric intake in a 24-hour period should not be affected in the least by fasting.

Unlike the workout plan where I gave several examples, I only have one example on the nutrition plan. Regardless of your goals, this nutrition plan will suit your needs and your body will settle into a natural weight when you couple this nutrition plan with a workout plan.

Remember, you need to eat in order to lose

weight. If you do not take in enough calories your body will eventually catch on to that and start to conserve its resources (fat stores) needed for immediate energy. So while you may see immediate results from dieting, those results will eventually taper off and stop for a while. If you continue to cut calories to try to lose weight, your body will eventually kick back into gear and actually start burning away muscle (which no one wants!) in order to save the fat stores for immediate needs. This leaves you with higher body fat percentage and a softer looking build. Make sure you eat enough of the *right* foods even when you are trying to lose weight. Keep your body satisfied and it will burn the fat that you want it to burn.

You can vary the amount of protein, carbs, and fat that you intake in this nutrition plan, but other than that everything remains the same. It's all about protein, good carbs (no sugar), and good fats. If you stick to these basic principles you will find that your body will settle into a natural, healthy weight. I like to use my protein as my variable as most of the fat I intake is tied directly to the protein. I eat a lot, but it is over 90% meats and veggies. This has no negative impact on my build no matter how much I eat. I try to stick to that 0.5g-1.0g of protein per pound of body weight. Even if I drop down around 0.5g I don't see much weight loss. Conversely, if I up that intake to 1.0g+ I do see some muscle gain, but nothing crazy. My body has found its optimal weight. In the last eight years I have not been below 190-lbs or higher than 200-lbs.

My last comment on eating is don't look for excuses to cheat. Like I said, I certainly indulge at times, but I don't look for reasons to do so. If you try hard enough you can always find a reason, like an anniversary, birthday, holiday, it's Friday. But there will *always* be a birthday, anniversary, holiday and, I am pretty sure, a Friday. If you look hard enough you will always find an excuse to eat junk. Stick to your plan. You will be glad you did every time you look in a mirror.

Chapter 7

Supplementation

Supplementing can be very complex and very expensive. The supplements you choose are going to be dependent on the results you are trying to achieve. There are pre-workout boosters, intra-workout supplements, post-workout supplements, every day supplements, weight loss supplements, muscle building supplements, joint supplements, and cognitive function supplements. Some people will use all of these or a combination of them. There is no right or wrong answer as to exactly what or how many supplements you should use. You really need to set your goals and experiment with supplements in order to determine the effect and whether or not you are getting the results that you desire. Once you determine that, you can define the supplements that you should be using.

My philosophy on supplementing is to keep it very simple. It is a fact that we need to supplement on some level to gain real results. But with my current goals I like to put as few man-made products into my body as possible, so the supplements I use are derived naturally. I have experimented a lot with supplementation over the years. I have tried various fat burners, pre-workout supplements, intra-workout supplements, post-workout supplements, creatine, proteins, etc. I have done everything but steroids. While I have seen moderate gains with everything that I used, I am now down to using just three items and have seen more gain over the last six months than I have in the last six years.

Krill Oil

I now take Antarctic Krill Oil tablets. I take 1000mg per day (in the morning). I feel that these have really helped my joints, which is important to me as I age. I also feel this supplement has actually helped in the muscle building process. As it says in its literature, if krill is good enough to sustain the largest mammals on earth it should be good enough for you.

You can increase the amount you take of this if you choose. I have taken double this amount for a period of time and I know other people who take up to 3000mg per day. For me, I have found that 1000mg has been effective and I have not found it worth taking more than that. With any supplement you take you should experiment with the dosage and determine what an optimal amount is for you.

MCT Oil

MCT stands for medium chain triglycerides and these are derived from coconut oil (which I also use quite liberally). I have read a lot about MCT oil recently and all of the great benefits. If you look at the nutrition label it consists of all fat. So seemingly one would look at this and think it is unhealthy, but you would be wrong. Fat consisting of MCT's is not broken down and stored in the body the same way as bad fats. Actually, the body takes the MCT's and uses them kind of like a carbohydrate substitute (energy source) so it actually promotes the burning of fat in your body. I like to take two tablespoons of this in my coffee in the morning, about 30 minutes prior to my workout. I have noticed increased energy in my workout and that I have been shedding body fat.

Protein

I will also use supplements to achieve my required amount of protein intake, because it is really difficult to take in 200g of protein without any supplementation. Not only do you have to eat a lot of food, but it is difficult to find the time to prepare it as well. I have a hard time digesting the amount of food needed to intake that much protein, spaced out far enough so that you actually get all the benefits. Therefore, I supplement several times per day with either a protein bar or protein shake. It is only protein and nothing else. I do not take a mass builder or meal replacement shakes/bars or anything similar. I like to keep it very clean and simple. I will use whey protein mixed with water or almond milk, or a peanut butter protein bar. I also have a casein protein on hand. I use the casein if I find myself supplementing at night, as casein is a slower processing protein that works well while you sleep. I take a protein supplement one or two times per day, which gets me 30-60g of protein and helps me to hit my goal of 200g per day. The only down side to protein supplements is that they do contain a small amount of sugar (usually less than 10g) and you know by now how I feel about sugar. But in this case I feel the benefit of the 30-60g of protein is worth the sugar intake.

I take the protein supplements strictly to get protein into my body to help with the muscle building. I will buy protein bars that I can easily carry with me wherever I go to eat as a snack between meals or in some cases as a meal substitute if I have no other choice.

Supplements should be used to supplement already great eating habits. You aren't going to drink your way to an additional 25 lbs of lean muscle by downing protein shakes. You need to get your main protein from animals and add in supplements here and there. Just like your eating, you should also try to stay consistent with the supplements that you take. Your body needs time to adjust to certain supplements and you will want to make sure that you are not missing workouts because you feel ill from the effects of your supplements.

Just like with my workout and nutrition plans, my approach with supplementation is simple, sustainable, and affordable. Using just these few supplements will not get you built like a body builder, but you will notice some very positive benefits. As you get stronger and advance to more aggressive goals, you will need to increase the intensity of your workout and really up your supplement intake to include stacking of supplements. This is something I may consider experimenting with in the near future, but for long-term day-to-day use I would recommend sticking with a few base supplements.

Chapter 8

Consistency

Consistency is one of the most important aspects of your routine. I am referring to the consistency in both your workout and your nutrition plan. Remember, the key elements for my approach is to develop a plan for yourself that is: 1.) Consistent and 2.) sustainable (which we will discuss in the next chapter). Habits are derived from consistency in whatever you do. We need to focus on positive things such as working out and proper eating habits, while doing these things consistently and forming habits around them.

Workout Consistency

When I refer to consistency in the workout I am not referring to doing the exact same workout over and over again. You should vary your workout for sure as discussed in Chapter 4. The consistency is the cycle in which you work out and the time of day you work out.

In my opinion, the time of day you work out is extremely important. I feel there are a lot of benefits to working out first thing in the morning. First of all, it promotes discipline, the need to get out of bed and get to the gym. You will find that this will begin to set the tone for your day. Despite expending a ton of energy working out, you will feel a boost in energy throughout the day from this early morning workout. Second, you can take advantage of six to eight hours of fasting (during sleep), which takes no effort or discipline to achieve. If you recall from Chapter 5, there are a lot of benefits to working out on an empty stomach and if you do your workout in the morning it eliminates the need for you to do dedicated fasting prior to your workout.

Now, even though I am partial to early morning workouts, I understand that may not work for everybody. So regardless of what time of day you want to work out, just make sure you try to maintain consistency with the time of day. This will help you to stay focused on your workout routine and promote staying with it and getting your workout in. Also, by maintaining a consistent time each day it will help you to plan when to eat and make it easier to get your couple hours of fasting in prior to your workout.

For consistency in your workout cycle you should make sure you define the work/rest schedule that you are going to follow and stick to it for a period of time (at least one month). In my example, I go longer for parts of my cycle (up to three months), but do a routine for as little as one month. Just don't be jumping around. If you are going to work out three days and rest one day, then do that for an extended period of time before changing it up.

Nutrition Consistency

I touched on the consistency aspect of eating just briefly in the nutrition section. Maintaining consistency is the most difficult aspect of your nutrition plan because of all of the outside distractions (i.e. birthdays, anniversaries, etc.) which may prevent you from maintaining your eating habits. You should build your plan around healthy sustainable eating habits and stick to it. Just remember that you want to eat right 90% of the time. If you do this, you will likely find yourself eating healthy nearly 100% of the time as this promotes constant thought about what you eat and if you strive for that percentage of achieving healthy eating habits it won't allow for cheating on a weekly (or more frequent) basis.

Another thing that you must do is that you need to learn to enjoy the foods that are healthy for you and embrace the process of preparing this food. When cooking fresh foods, it takes a little knowledge and work to bring out the flavor you want. I am not a fan of diet plans that have you eating plain, bland foods just for the nutritional value. I want you to enjoy eating like I do! If you take some time to learn a little about cooking and embrace the process, you will find it easy to follow your plan and maintain your consistency. As a little added bonus, when you prepare a meal well and really enjoy the flavors it is a very rewarding experience.

No matter what you are doing in life, consistency is the key to success. We are simply applying it to maintaining our healthy lifestyle. Staying consistent with your workout and eating habits is difficult so I recommend focusing on the results. Get your joy from the *results* of the work you put in....this is the reward. Don't look at a day off from the gym as a reward or some big dessert as a reward. Your result is what is rewarding! People noticing your effort and changes in your body is rewarding! If you take the small bits of advice in this chapter, you will find that maintaining a consistent workout is achievable.

Chapter 9

Sustainability

Once you establish a consistent workout and diet, the next step is to ensure that it is sustainable. Remember, you should not be focused on short-term achievements. You want a long-term plan with long-term results. This is about living a lifestyle not just achieving some short term goal by losing some weight that you will gain right back. I want you to be able to live this way indefinitely without burning out and quitting!

Sustainable Workout

When you develop your workout plan you want to make sure you are creating something that you can do over the long haul. And you want to switch up your workout with some amount of frequency so you don't get bored. Combating burn-out is a very important aspect of working out and burn-out can happen for several reasons. We will discuss what I think the top three reasons are for people getting burnt out.

One of those reasons is simply getting bored with your routine as you find yourself doing the same things over and over again. As I mentioned in my workout section, I like to vary the exercises and the weight/rep ratio throughout my workout cycle. I prefer to do a four-month cycle (three months of heavier weight/low rep and one month of low weight/high rep work). Even within this cycle, I vary the exercises and intensity weekly. I also like to vary my cardio. For a long time I just ran for my cardio, but now I find myself running, biking, using machines (stepper, elliptical, rower, etc.), doing Jiu-Jitsu, CrossFit, or other class work. Variety keeps things interesting and keeps you engaged in your program.

Another reason people get burned-out is they can't sustain the level of intensity of the workout program they develop. A lot of folks jump into a workout routine and go crazy with the level of intensity. Having a workout that is too intense can also lead to injury. When creating a workout plan you really need to walk a fine line in terms of the intensity or weight/reps you use. During your average daily workout you should not be working at your absolute maximum effort. While you should definitely up the intensity on occasion and go to failure, you should not do this day in and day out. You will begin to dread going to the gym and risk injury if you think you need to work out with that level of intensity all of the time.

The last reason that I see for people burning out is that they are disappointed with the pace of the results. Remember back to Chapter 3 where I mentioned working out isn't quick, fun, or easy neither are your results. But you do want them to be sustainable. Think of it like easy come, easy go. If you see quick gains, you will lose those gains quickly as well. Be patient as you measure your results and stay focused on the long-term results.

Sustainable Diet

This one is extremely important and very tough to accomplish. Just like the workout, we want to make sure that we can continue healthy eating habits so we can see long-term results. When you create your diet, just like the workout, you don't want to make it too extreme. If you find that you are depriving yourself of everything this will lead to you craving those bad foods that provide instant, temporary gratification.

Your diet should consist of a balance of protein,

good carbs, and good fats. If you give yourself all of these elements in your diet you'll be able to eat a lot of different foods and have a very satisfying diet to help with combating cravings. Again, you simply need to focus on eating healthy 90% of the time.

Chapter 10

Discipline vs. Motivation

This chapter is dedicated to the one thing that can keep you going and on track with your workout and diet: discipline. Discipline is simply having the intestinal fortitude to do the tough things, like eating right or working out, in the face of the temptation to give up on your commitment. It is doing the things you have to do even when you don't want to do them. This chapter is what it is all about! If you can only take one thing out of this book then rip out this chapter, and burn the rest of the book. If you can implement discipline in your life, then you will figure out the rest. Discipline will give you what you need to execute once you decide what you want to do with your life. Discipline will get you results and keep you going forever.

Many fitness "experts" talk about motivation. Group workout classes that are competitive, like CrossFit, play on this motivation tactic. But what happens when you don't have the group to

104

motivate you? Is that what you really need to push you through your workout? Or will you be able to compartmentalize and be disciplined when you find yourself working out alone?

For some folks motivation is seasonal. They want to look good in a bathing suit or for a wedding or some other special event. I know so many people who will take this approach and for a short period of time they will be ultra-dedicated. They will lose weight, get in shape, and feel great then when the event comes and goes they go right back to their old habits. While this type of motivation can most definitely help you in the short-term, it will not help you to stay in the game for the long-term. Everything that motivates you has an end. You will eventually get to the event that you were striving for, then what? Will you find something else to motivate you? Chances are you will eventually find something that will motivate you for another short period of time or, in extreme cases, nothing will come along. Then you won't have any motivation and you will find yourself spiraling into being fat and out of shape.

It's important not to confuse motivation with goals. Goals can often be perceived as motivators because you can use a goal, such as weight loss, to motivate you toward achieving that goal. And I don't want you to think I am contradicting myself because I devoted a chapter early on to goal setting. I don't like to think of goals as motivation. Rather I like to use goals as markers to measure progress then readjust those goals upward as they are reached. Goals should be used to achieve continuous improvement.

Instead of identifying things that motivate you and relying on motivation to push you to work out, I would like to challenge you to try a new approach. Be disciplined! Treat your workout and diet as a way of life and something you *have to do* to achieve your desired lifestyle. Then do it each and every day. Don't make excuses, don't skip days, don't let weakness creep in and prevent you from doing your workout. Be disciplined and do what you need to do even when you don't want to do it. Anyone can go to the gym or for a run when it is convenient. Doing it when you don't want to do it, when you are tired, sick, injured, or sore that is what's hard and that's what separates you from the pack and gets you the results. Remember, if it were easy everyone would do it.

You are probably thinking, "I am not disciplined, so how do I become disciplined?" This is easy-- you just do it. Just be disciplined. This is simply a matter of waking up one day and saying I want to do this, then executing it day in and day out WITHOUT FAIL. I can say this because I have done it. Before I made the decision to change my lifestyle eight years ago I was overweight, out of shape, and just plain lazy. I was the complete opposite of disciplined. And I am not just talking about my fitness, I am talking about my entire life. I didn't strive for anything better in my career, I didn't do anything extra around the house, I didn't go to the gym, I didn't do anything. I simply existed and consumed, which was no way to live.

I finally made the decision one day that I was going to turn it all around and I implemented discipline in every aspect of my life, but it all started with diet and exercise. You will see that once you begin exercising, you will discover that discipline is not something that you can (or will want to) just shut off. I became disciplined in everything. At work it was noticeable as I was finishing up required assignments ahead of schedule and with a high level of quality, I enrolled for my MBA and completed it in 15 months, I was spending more time with my wife and kids, and at home nothing went unfinished. Being disciplined became almost a compulsion, like an obsession. I had a sense of urgency about everything that I did. It didn't matter if it was the most important or most trivial of tasks. A task was a task and needed to be completed and I took it upon myself to complete those tasks as quickly and effectively as possible. Start your discipline with your nutrition and workout and you will see how it rolls over and improves the rest of your life.

<u>Chapter 11</u>

Why Should I Do This?

You may be asking yourself at this point, "Why should I do all of this?" The answer is simple........you should do this for you! There are so few things in this world that you have 100% control over. Your level of fitness is one of those things. I am not one of those people who believe that you can do whatever you want no matter what you put your mind to, that's unrealistic thinking. Some people may be limited in their physical or mental capacity, but for the most part no matter where you come from, how much money you have, how much time you have, your height, weight, financial position, or physical handicap, there is *something* you can do to improve your physical state. Improving your physical condition gives you freedom to do so many things that would have otherwise seemed out of reach. Think about how many times you want to do something and think to yourself, "I can't do that." Now, imagine never having to tell yourself that again. Imagine having the confidence to take on anything that is physically put in front of you and having the ability to do it.

In addition, your cognitive function will be vastly improved with proper nutrition and exercise. I can speak firsthand to this. Since incorporating all of these things into my life I cannot believe how much my mind has improved. My memory is better, I speak clearer, I present better in front of others; the results have just been tremendous. Again, I can't speak to the science of it in this book; the benefits from the nutrients from food or endorphins released from exercise, but you can easily research it and draw your own conclusions. What I can tell you is exactly what I have experienced, which is tremendous gains in the area of cognitive function with no supplementation targeting that direct result.

A healthy nutrition and regular exercise plan have been shown to slow the effects of aging. Now please note, I said it has shown to slow the *effects of aging*, not stop the aging process or reverse the aging process. But you can delay the process with proper nutrition and exercise. This evidence is undisputable. If you look at people who work out regularly, have healthy eating habits, and limit their exposure to the sun (I

110

threw that in there because that's a killer on aging....doesn't necessarily pertain to this book, but will make you age like crazy) they look 10 years younger than people who do nothing. You can't control all aspects of aging; people get gray hair, lose their hair, and develop wrinkles. But you can control how you feel physically. A good nutrition plan and workout plan will keep your muscles toned, your heart healthy and, if you don't overdo it, your joints will also hold up better.

Proper diet and exercise have been shown to improve your overall feeling of happiness and to combat depression. There can be several factors that are speculated to drive this result, such as the nutrients and the chemical impact on your brain or body. I am someone who has done this and I will say the better that you feel and the more comfortable you are with your body, the happier you will be with yourself and others. Being healthy, feeling good, and looking good are not mutually exclusive goals so if you are striving to do one, chances are that the others are going to fall into place. Let's be honest, the better you look the better you feel, the more confidence you have! Once you can get happy with yourself the sky is truly the limit in what you can do.

Chapter 12

Summary & Conclusion

I hope you enjoyed this book and took some valuable and useful information from what I have written, and have been able to understand the basic principles. If you take nothing else from this book, at least follow these few steps in detail. I think you will be happy with the results.

1) Make a choice about your lifestyle
    a. How do you want to live?
    b. What do you want to look like?
    c. What do you want to be capable of doing?
    d. What kind of activity level do you want to have?

2) Set your goals
    a. Our primary goal is overall fitness, but what goals, such as weight loss, body composition, weight

lifting, cardio, etc. are you going to use as markers to get there?

b. Don't take too much time to celebrate. Hit your goal, readjust it up, and get after the new goal!

3) Fitness isn't easy, quick, or fun, so get over it
   a. Fitness is not easy.
   b. Getting fit takes time, lots of time, so be patient.
   c. Fitness is not fun all the time.
   d. Don't look for things you like or things that are quick or things that are easy. In fitness and in life you will never see results pursuing anything this way, so just get over it, buckle down, and get fit.

4) Develop a workout plan
   a. Get a game plan and go after it.
   b. I gave some examples.....there is no right or wrong answer, just get a plan.
   c. As you progress then you can tweak the plan to your needs.

5) Nutrition Plan
   a. Eat lots of protein and good fats.
   b. ELIMINATE sugar.
   c. Eat complex carbs.
   d. Make sure you are eating enough.....under-eating can have a detrimental effect
   e. Fasting - go long periods without eating (at least 12 hours), but make sure in the other 12 hours you are eating enough so you get adequate proteins, fats, and carbs.

6) Supplementation
   a. You need to supplement.
   b. At a minimum take the following:
      i. Krill Oil
      ii. MCT Oil
      iii. Protein
   c. Add supplements as you see fit, but use the above as a minimum.

7) Consistency
   a. Make sure that you are consistent in your workout and diet.
   b. Develop a plan and stick to your cycle.

8) Sustainability
   a. You should be able to continue with your routine forever.
   b. Remember not to burn yourself out:
      i. Design your workout so it is extremely difficult, but not impossible.
      ii. Design your nutrition plan so it is strict, but not insane.

9) Discipline
   a. Discipline is the KEY TO IT ALL!!!
   b. Just do what you need to do and do it for you.
   c. Do not rely on any motivation to get you to your goals.....only discipline.

As you think about everything in this book focus on the principles discussed – choosing your lifestyle, setting goals, discipline, consistency, and sustainability. I gave specific examples as a reference, but feel free to build your own plan around these basic principles. My intent was not to tell you exactly what to do, but to give you these very basic principles that I have found valuable so you can implement them in your own life.

I want to encourage you, no matter your current physical condition, to take that leap and commit to living a healthier lifestyle. You only get one chance at this life so why not live it to the fullest. Make your health and fitness a priority in your life. I have never heard anyone express any regret about getting healthier or fitter! Making that initial decision to start can be scary; don't be intimidated and let the fear of starting something new and unfamiliar hold you back. Live a life without fear! Make the decision to invest in your own well-being, take control, be disciplined, and NEVER give up on your goals! It will be hard, it will take time, and you will feel like quitting along the way, but I promise you that if you stick with it this will be the best decision you have ever made!

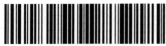

Made in the USA
Middletown, DE
24 July 2017